BELIEVE
in
Katie Lynn

By Bartholomew Resta, M.D.

Illustrated by Kitty Harvill

For my friend —

Believe in Esmé!

Bartholomew Resta MD

Eggman Publishing, Inc.
NASHVILLE, TENNESSEE

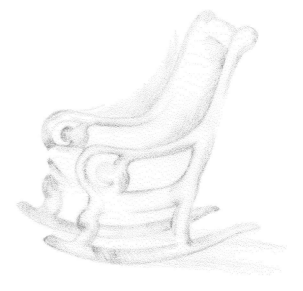

Text copyright © 1995 by Bartholomew Resta, M.D.
Illustrations © 1995 by Kitty Harvill

All rights reserved. No part of this publication may be reproduced or transmitted in any form or by any means, electronic or mechanical, including photocopy, recording, or any information storage and retrieval system, without permission in writing from the publisher.

Published by Eggman Publishing, Inc.
2909 Poston Avenue, Suite 203
Nashville, Tennessee 37203
(615) 327-9390
1-800-396-4626

Printed and bound in the United States of America

ISBN 1-886371-10-5
LOC 94-062209

Cover illustration by Kitty Harvill

Design, typography, and text production by Harvill Ross Studios Ltd., Little Rock, Arkansas

Scripture quotations are from the New Revised Standard Version of the Bible. Verses on page 3 represent 1 Corinthians 13:7–8. The selection on page 48 is from Matthew 25:40.

The hymn quoted on pages 24 and 46 is known as "The Welsh Lullaby," or "All Through the Night." The author is unknown, and the hymn is in the public domain.

FIRST EDITION

Written for Kathleen Francis.

This book is dedicated to three Mommies: Margaret, Catherine, and Peg.

LOVE
Bears all things, believes all things,
Hopes all things, endures all things.
Love never ends.

Many years ago, in a big hospital, a tiny baby was born. Her name was Katie Lynn. Katie was a *preemie* baby, born before she was ready for the world.

The doctors and nurses were afraid Katie was too small. They rushed her from the delivery room. "Out of our way!" they shouted. "We have a sick little baby here!"

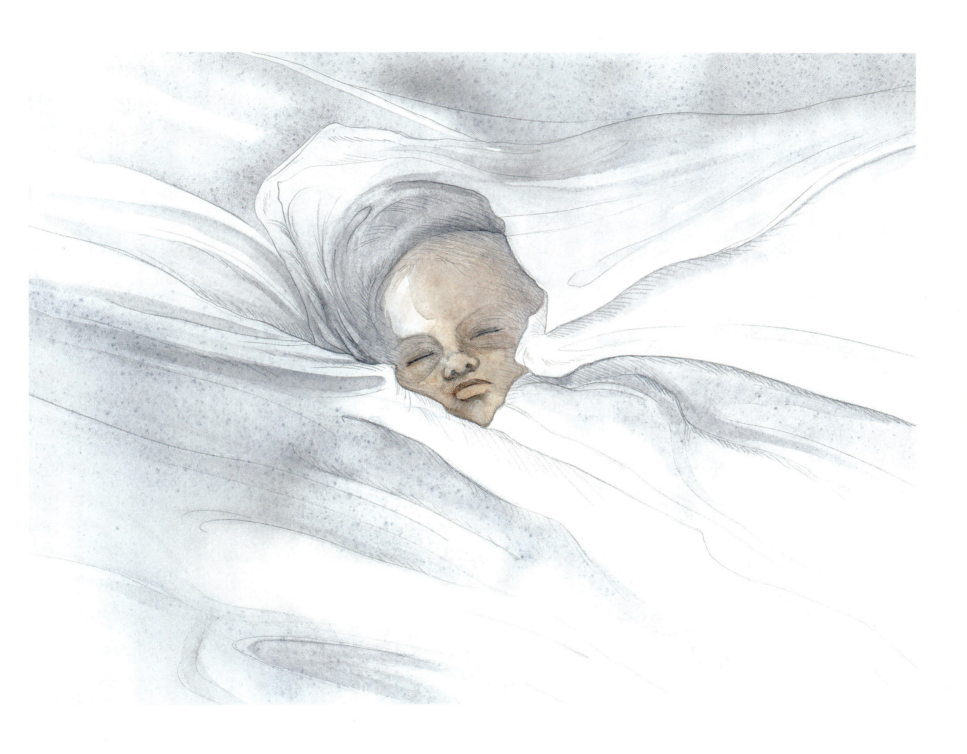

Mommy heard them and began to cry. Katie Lynn was the only family she had. She couldn't be sick! She had to get well!

In the room for sick babies, Katie's nurse weighed her. "Just two and a half pounds!" she called out. She carefully laid her on Bed One. Then, Katie stopped breathing!

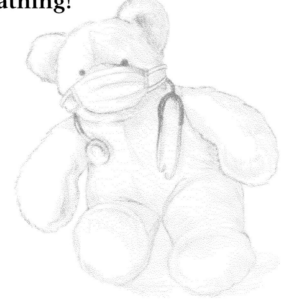

People came running to help. Quickly, a doctor put a tube in Katie's mouth. The tube went to a bag that looked like a big black balloon. A nurse squeezed the bag, over and over again. The balloon bag was breathing for Katie Lynn!

Katie's nurse dried her in a warm blanket. Then she taped red, black, and white wires to her arms and legs. Katie's doctor connected tubes to give her medicine.

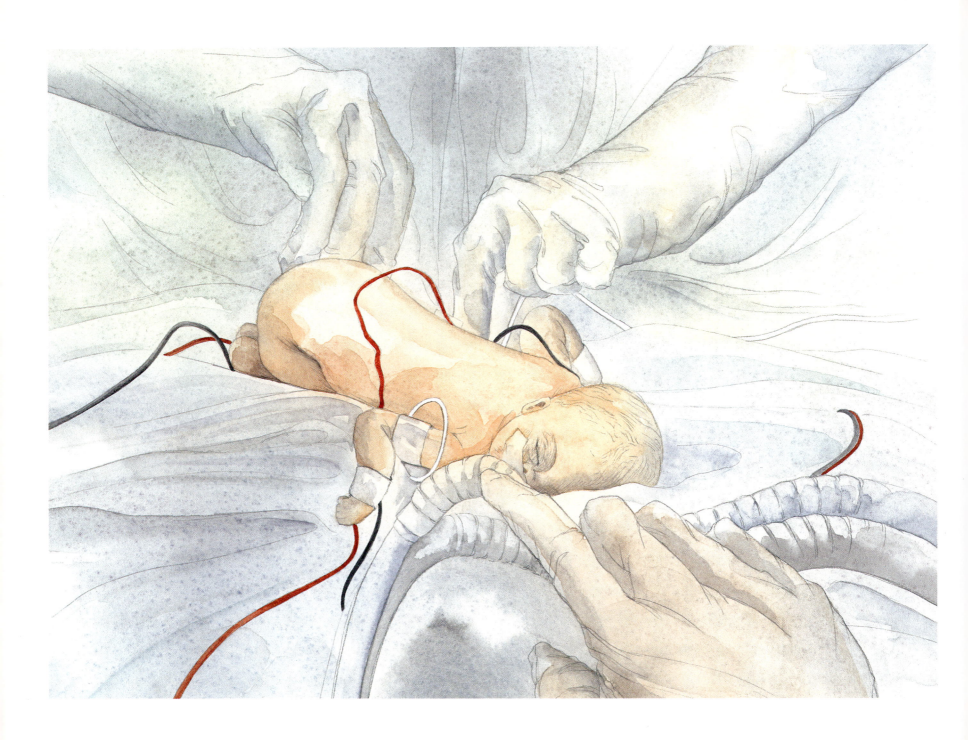

Every tube and wire went to a machine, and each machine made a noise if Katie needed something. ***Beep! Beep! Beep!*** told the nurses she needed water. A whistle blew if she was too cold. ***Clang! Clang! Clang!*** meant her heart had slowed down. Every noise brought helpers to Katie Lynn. They fussed over her till they solved the problem, then left till the next alarm.

Finally, Mommy got to visit. The doctor told her about Katie being sick. He told her about the medicine and the machines.

Even though the tubes and wires scared her, Mommy reached into Bed One and held Katie's hand.

"You mustn't do that," warned the doctor. "She is too small and too sick."

Mommy stopped. "May I stay with her?"

"Yes, but please don't touch."

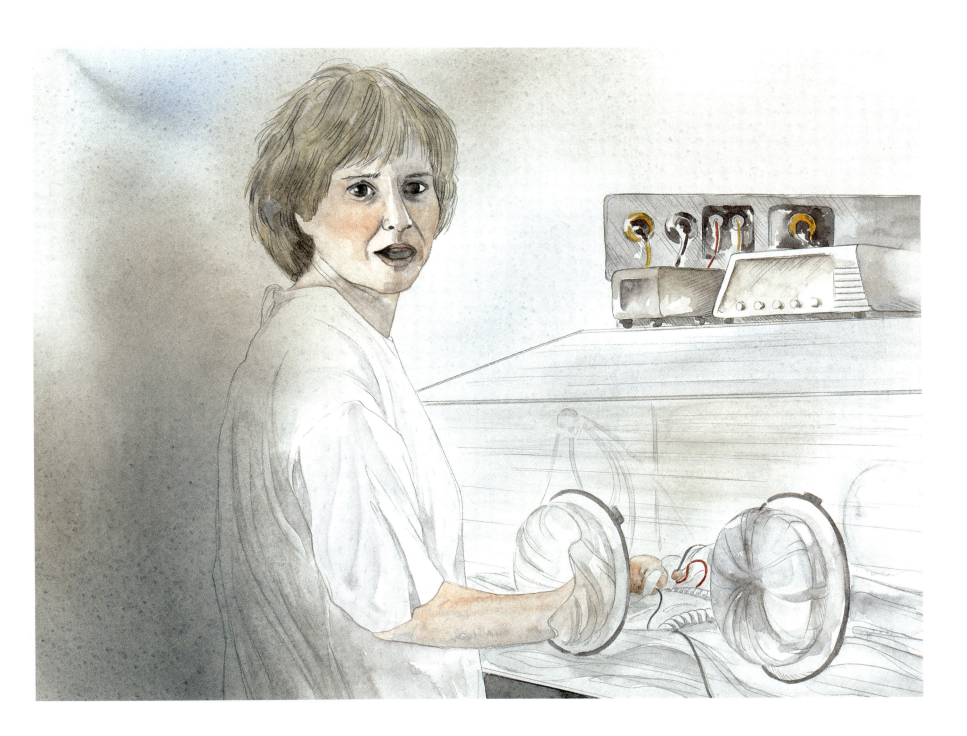

So Mommy sat down beside Katie Lynn. She stayed there day and night. Even though she couldn't touch Katie, Mommy never left her side.

Every morning, Katie's nurse weighed her. Then, the doctors came and talked about her. Instead of saying "Katie Lynn," they always called her "Bed One."

"Hmmm," Katie's doctor said. "Bed One has lost weight again. This is not good."

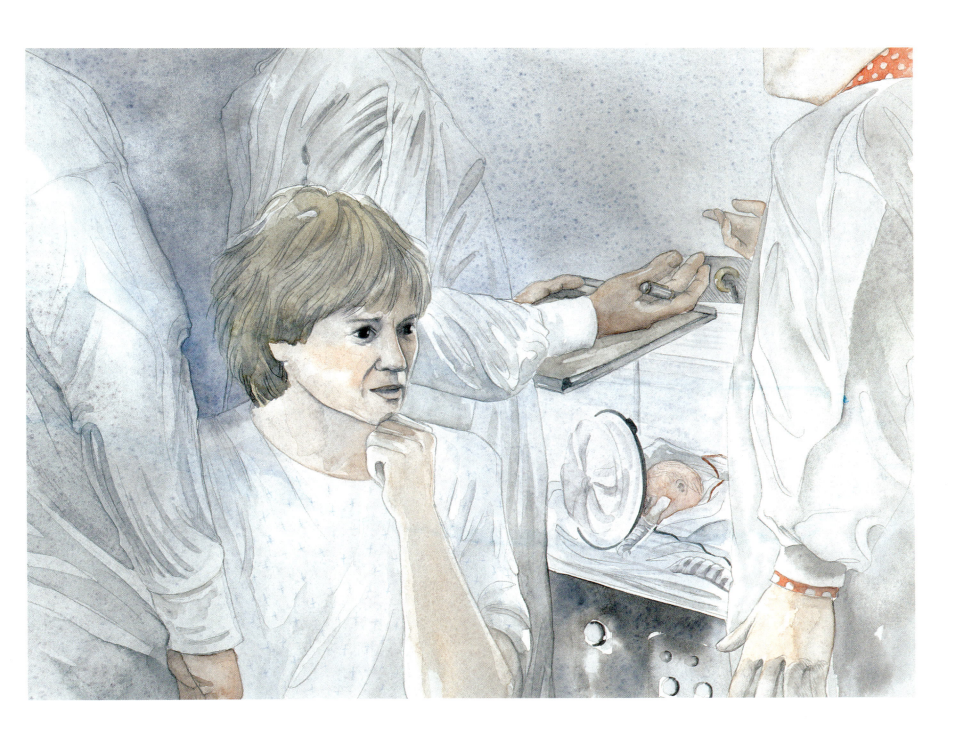

"Have you tried the new medicine for preemies? That will make Bed One grow!"

So they rolled in a new machine with the new medicine in it. The machine growled: ***Gurrrrh-urrrrh-urrrrh!***

Katie Lynn got smaller.

The doctors saw that the new medicine wasn't working.

"Have you heard about the new food for sick babies? That should make Bed One grow!"

So they hooked up a new machine to pump the new food. This machine was even noisier than the last. It groaned: ***Chunga-chunga-chunga!***

Katie kept getting smaller.

Soon, the doctors saw that the new food wasn't helping. "How about a bigger, better breathing machine? That might make Bed One grow!"

So the biggest machine yet rose up beside Katie. It roared: ***Whoosh-whoosh-whoosh!***

The machines never let up: ***Gurrrrh-urrrrh-urrrrh! Chunga-chunga-chunga! Whoosh-whoosh-whoosh!*** Alarms were always clanging. Bright lights shone day and night. Katie couldn't get any rest!

The machines piled higher and higher. Katie Lynn got smaller and smaller.

Finally one morning, all the doctors came to examine Katie. Mommy backed away as they crowded around Bed One. The doctors didn't see that Mommy was still there.

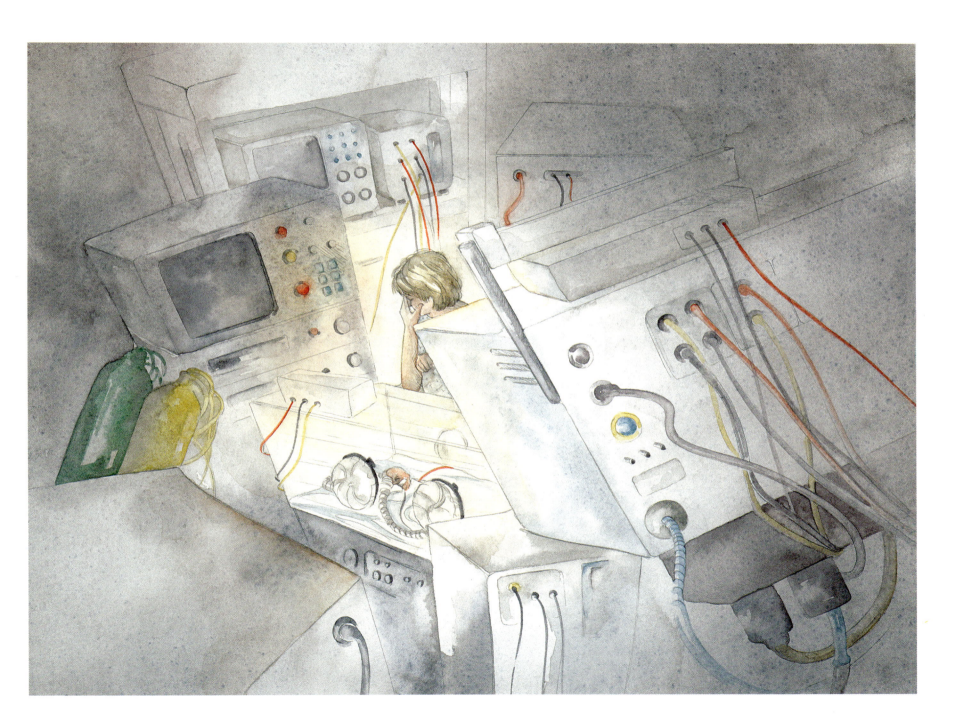

The doctors were sad. Preemie babies could have lots of problems. Katie Lynn seemed to have them all.

They whispered:

"I don't believe Bed One will ever breathe right. There is something wrong with her lungs," said the doctor with the bear on her stethoscope.

"I don't believe Bed One will ever see right. There is something wrong with her eyes," said the doctor with the big bow tie.

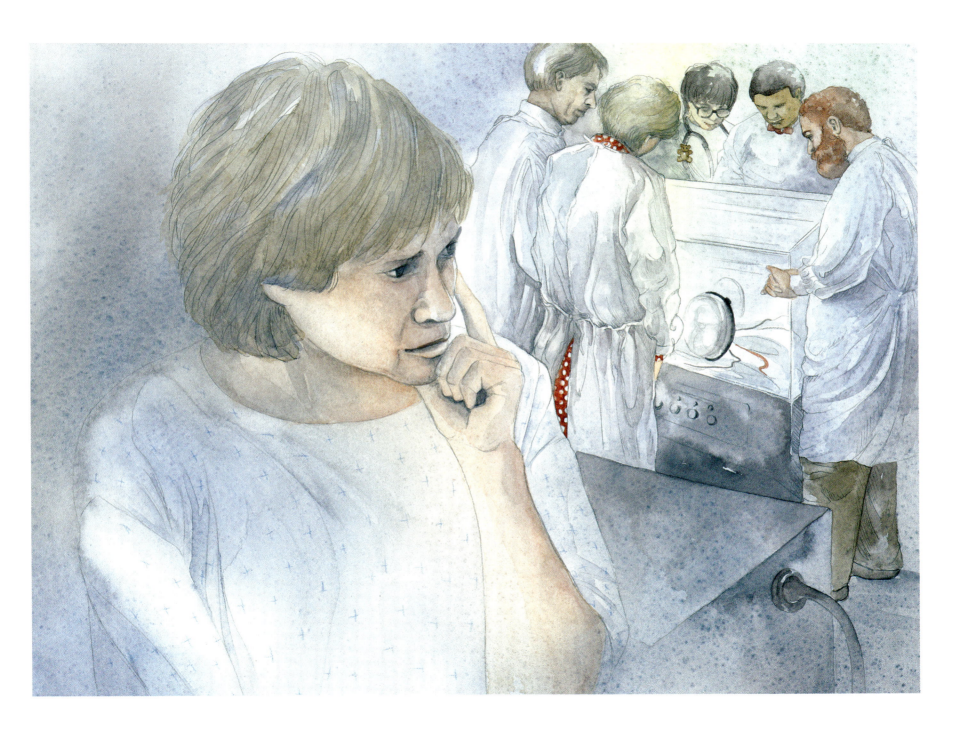

"I don't believe Bed One will ever hear right. There is something wrong with her ears," said the doctor in the polka dot dress.

"I don't believe Bed One will ever learn right. There is something wrong with her brain," said the doctor with the bushy red beard.

Then Katie's own doctor spoke, slowly and sadly. "I don't believe Bed One will ever grow right. I don't believe she will grow at all. In fact, I don't believe Bed One will be here tomorrow—unless a miracle happens."

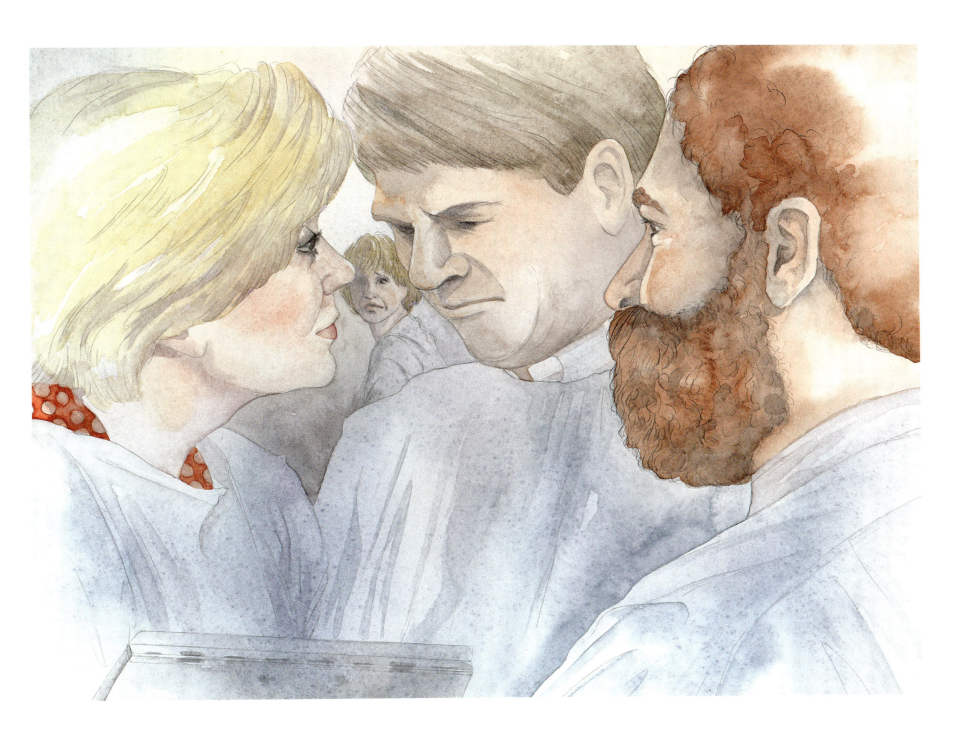

The doctors shook their heads and walked away.

Mommy heard everything the doctors said. All day she sat at Katie's side. All day she prayed that Katie would be with her tomorrow.

Katie's nurse saw that Mommy needed something special.

She brought a rocking chair for Mommy and hung curtains around it. She turned down the lights and the alarms. Gently, she lifted Katie from Bed One and placed her in Mommy's arms. Then, she left Katie and Mommy alone.

Mommy bundled up Katie, tubes and wires and all. She sat with her in the rocker and stroked her face.

"Little baby, sweet tiny baby! Your name is Katie Lynn, and I'm your Mommy."

"I believe in you, Katie Lynn. I will be with you and for you, always. I will not let you go."

Then, in a soft sweet voice, Mommy began to sing:

Sleep, my child, and peace attend thee,
All through the night;
Guardian angels God will send thee,
All through the night;

Soft the drowsy hours are creeping,
Hill and vale in slumber steeping,
I my loving vigil keeping,
All through the night.

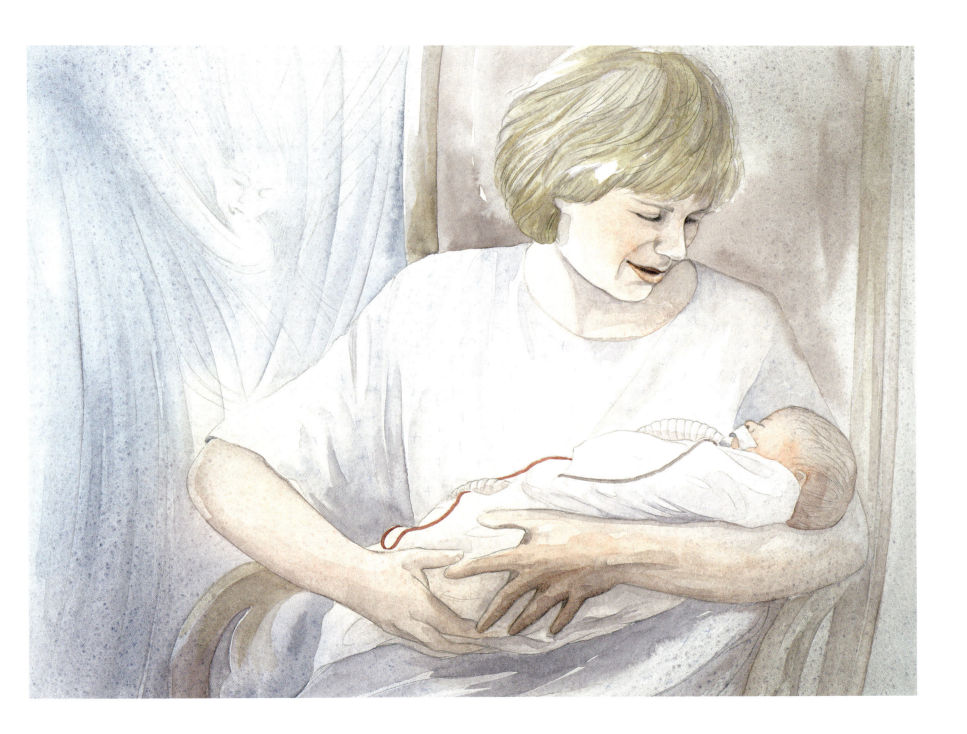

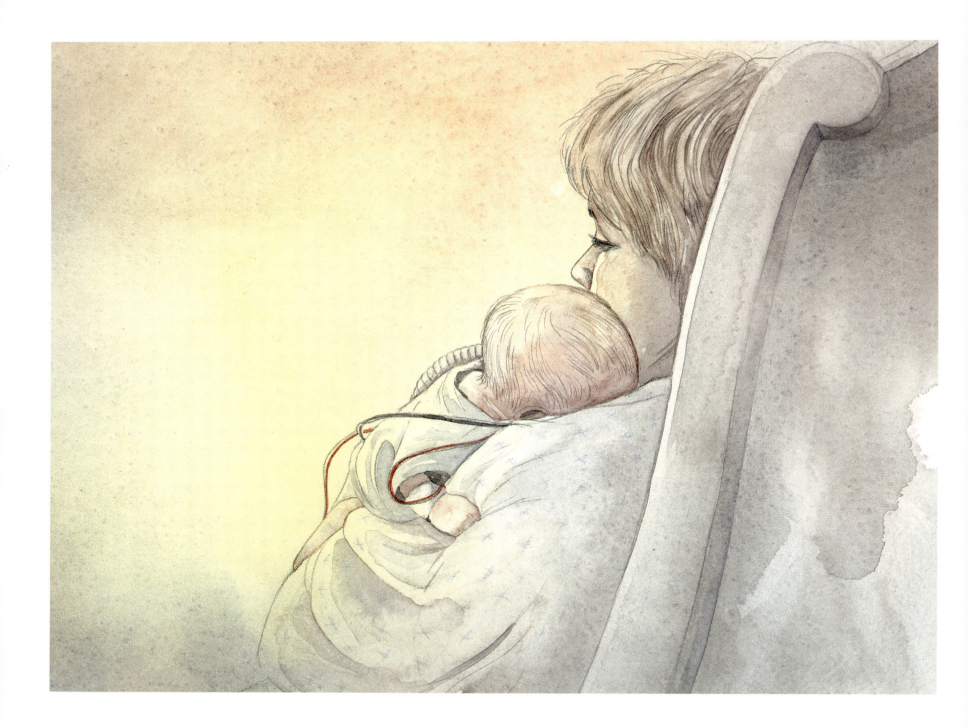

She rocked her baby and sang to her all night long. Katie nodded off to sleep in her mother's arms. Katie was able to rest.

Early next morning, Katie's nurse returned. She pulled back the curtains and smiled. She lifted Katie back into Bed One—but first, she weighed her.

Katie hadn't lost any weight!

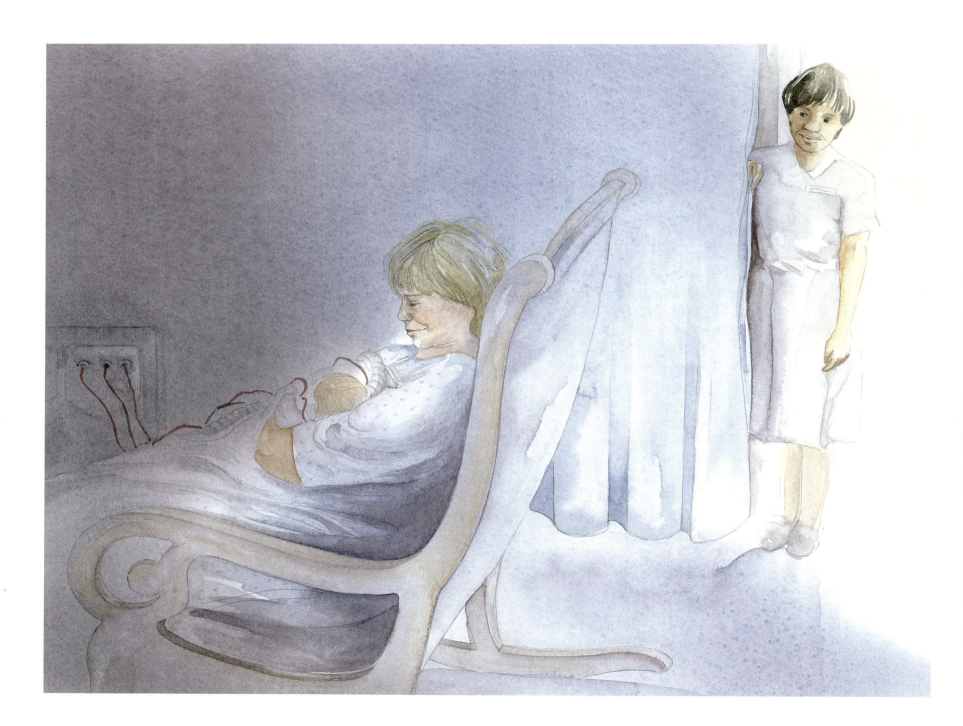

Her doctor examined Katie again. "I still don't believe Bed One will grow," he said.

That night, Katie's nurse brought back the rocking chair. Again she turned down the lights and the alarms.

Mommy cradled her little baby bundle. She whispered, "Your name is Katie Lynn. I believe in you!" Mommy rocked Katie and sang to her all night long.

In the morning, Katie's nurse weighed her.

She gained an ounce! Katie gained weight!

Every night, Mommy told her baby, "Your name is Katie Lynn. I believe in you!" Every morning, Katie weighed more.

Her doctor was puzzled. "Why is Bed One gaining weight? We aren't using any new machines or new medicines. Does anyone understand what is happening? What are we doing right?"

Katie's nurse spoke up. "I know that Katie's Mommy wasn't supposed to touch her. But when you said you didn't believe she would make it to another day . . ."

So Katie's nurse told them about turning down the lights and the alarms. She told them about Mommy holding Katie and rocking with her and singing to her. She told them about Mommy believing in Katie Lynn.

Katie's doctor thought and thought. "I believe we forgot the most important medicine of all. It's time for some changes here!"

They turned down the alarms, and they turned down the lights at night. Everyone began to talk and sing to Katie Lynn.

Her nurse made a sign for Katie's bed. It said,

"My name is Katie Lynn. Believe in me!"

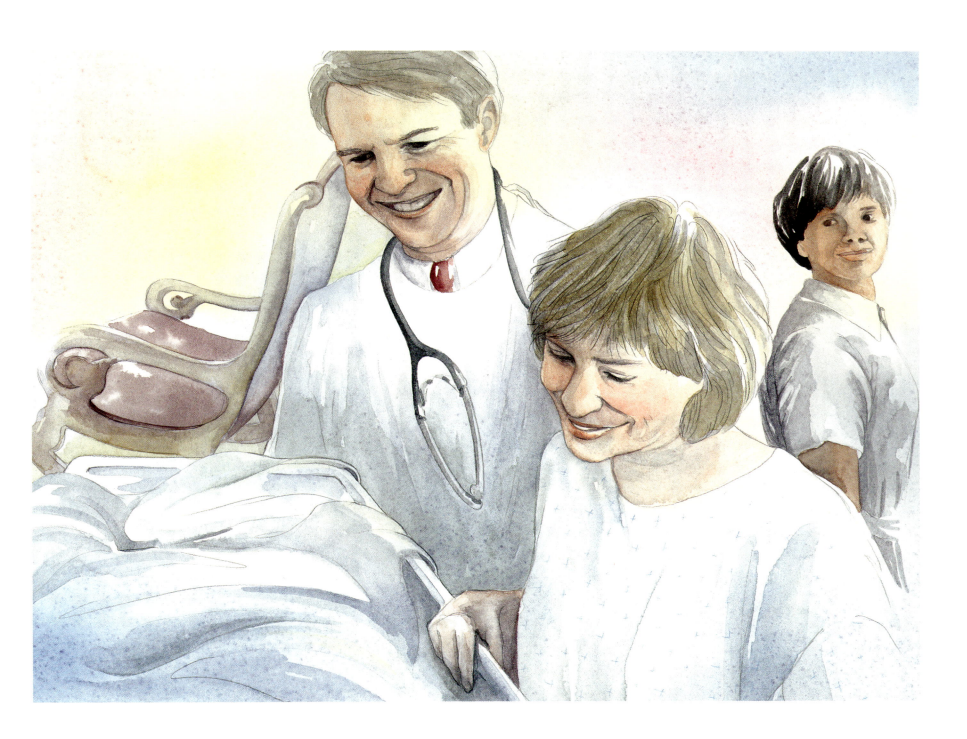

No one ever talked about Bed One again. Instead, they talked about Katie Lynn!

Soon, Katie began to breathe on her own. Then, she learned to drink from a bottle. Now the machines got smaller and smaller, while Katie grew and grew!

Finally the day came for Katie to leave the hospital. Her nurse and doctor waved good-bye: "Come back and visit, Katie Lynn. We'll take you out for pizza!"

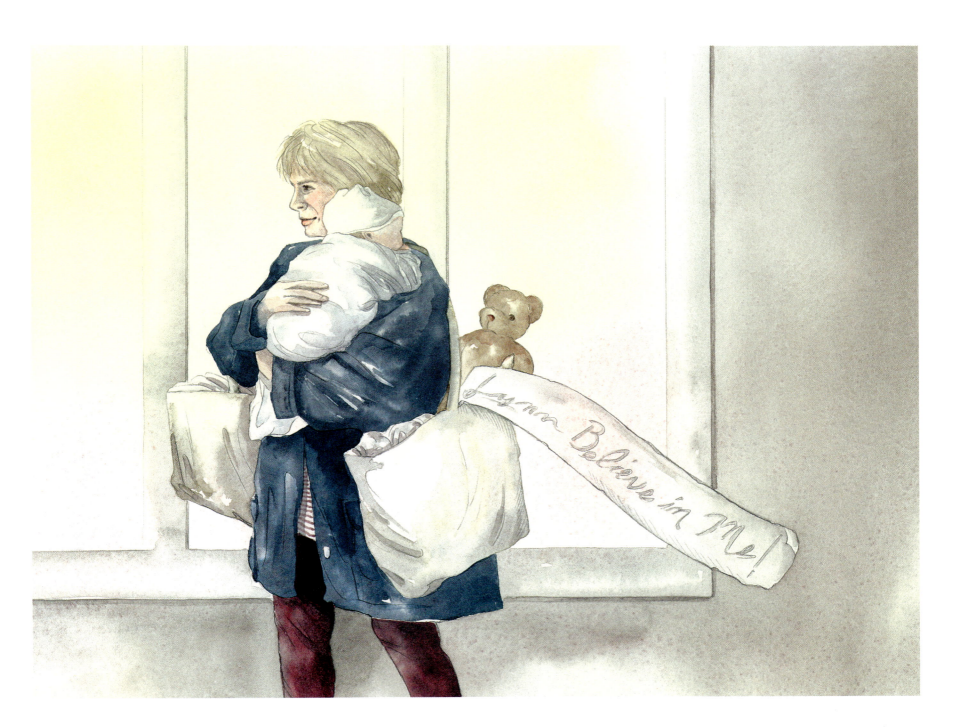

That night and every night, just like in the hospital, Mommy rocked her baby and sang to her. Every night she whispered, "Your name is Katie Lynn. I believe in you!" Katie heard those words so often that they echoed through her dreams.

Of course, Katie wasn't through with hospitals.

Since she had been a preemie baby, there was something different about her lungs. Sometimes she had trouble breathing. But Mommy believed in Katie Lynn. She took her back to the hospital. The doctor with the bear on her stethoscope gave Katie medicines so she could breathe better!

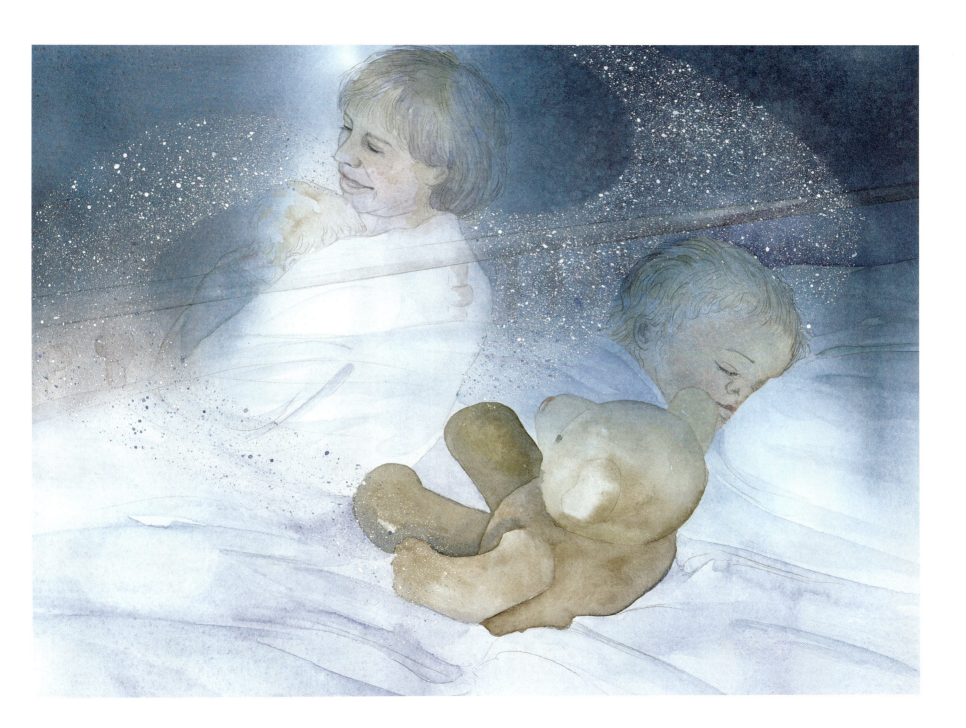

There was something different about Katie Lynn's eyes. She didn't see very well. But Mommy believed in Katie Lynn. The doctor with the big bow tie made glasses so she could see better!

There was something different about Katie Lynn's ears. She didn't hear very well. But Mommy believed in Katie Lynn. The doctor with the polka dot dress made a hearing aid so she could hear better!

And there was something different about Katie Lynn's brain. She had trouble learning. But by the time she was old enough to go to school, Katie Lynn believed in herself. The doctor with the bushy red beard showed her that she could learn well, if she took her time and studied carefully. So Katie Lynn did!

She studied as long as it took to learn whatever she wanted to learn. And she wanted to learn a lot!

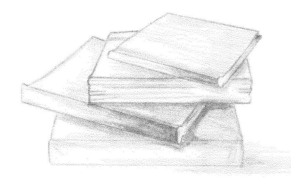

One year, after Katie had learned to read, she and Mommy returned to the room for sick babies. Katie looked in the window and saw a doctor and a nurse. They were both sitting in rocking chairs, cuddling little babies!

Katie read the signs on the beds:

"My name is James. Sing to me!"

"My name is Maggie. Hug me!"

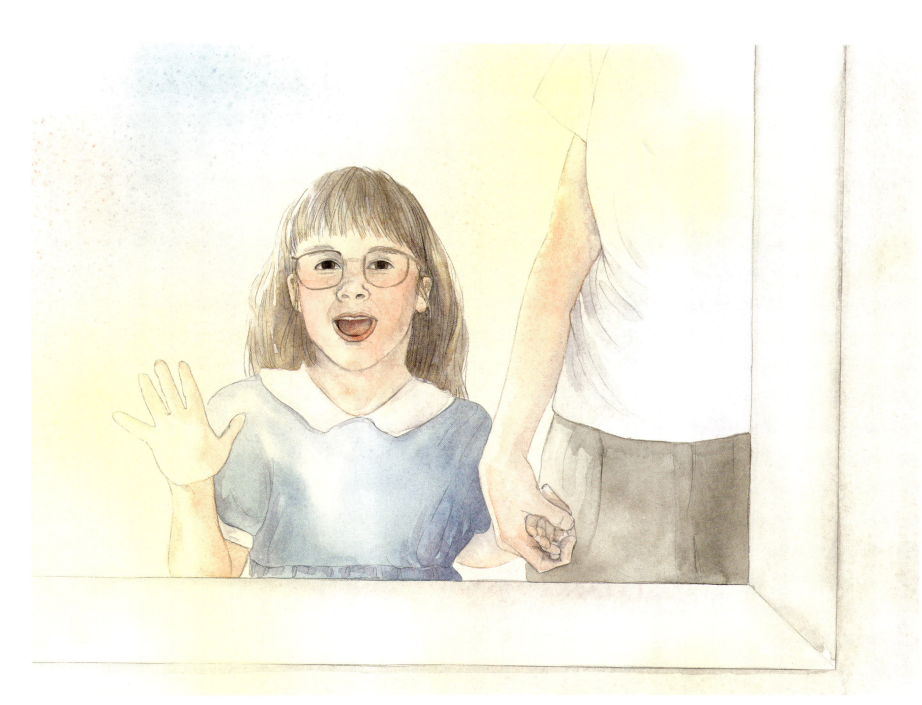

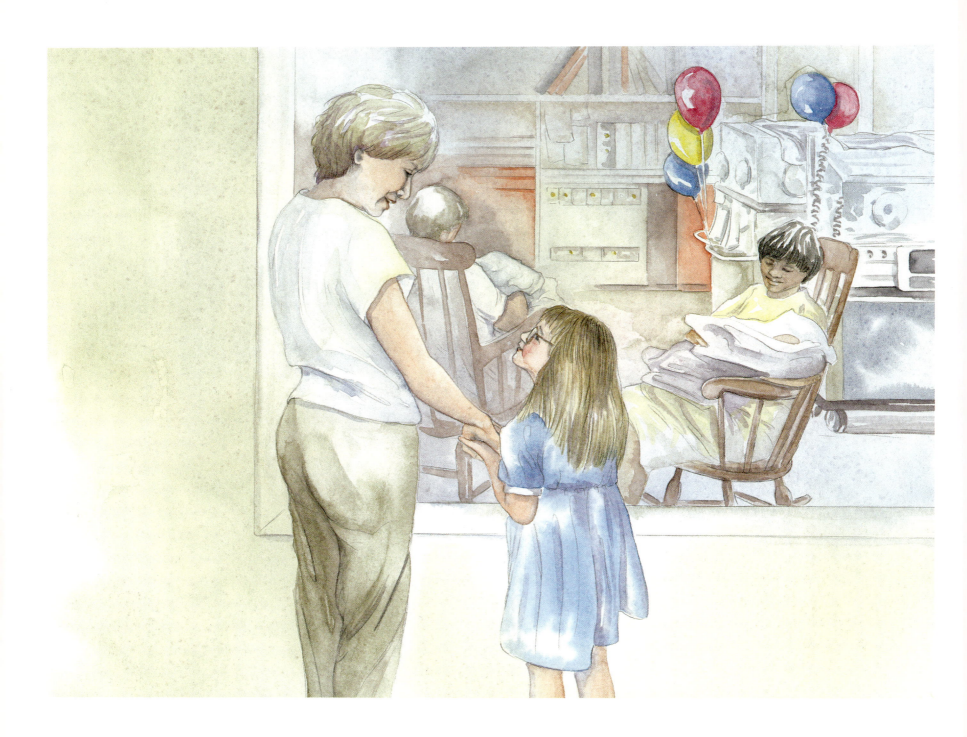

Katie thought that room was the neatest place she had ever seen. She told Mommy, "I'm going to do that when I grow up!"

Katie met her old doctor and her nurse. They were delighted to see how Katie had grown. They showed her the whole hospital. Then, they took her out for pizza!

Katie never forgot that day. She worked and worked and studied and studied. When she got older, she went to college and studied more.

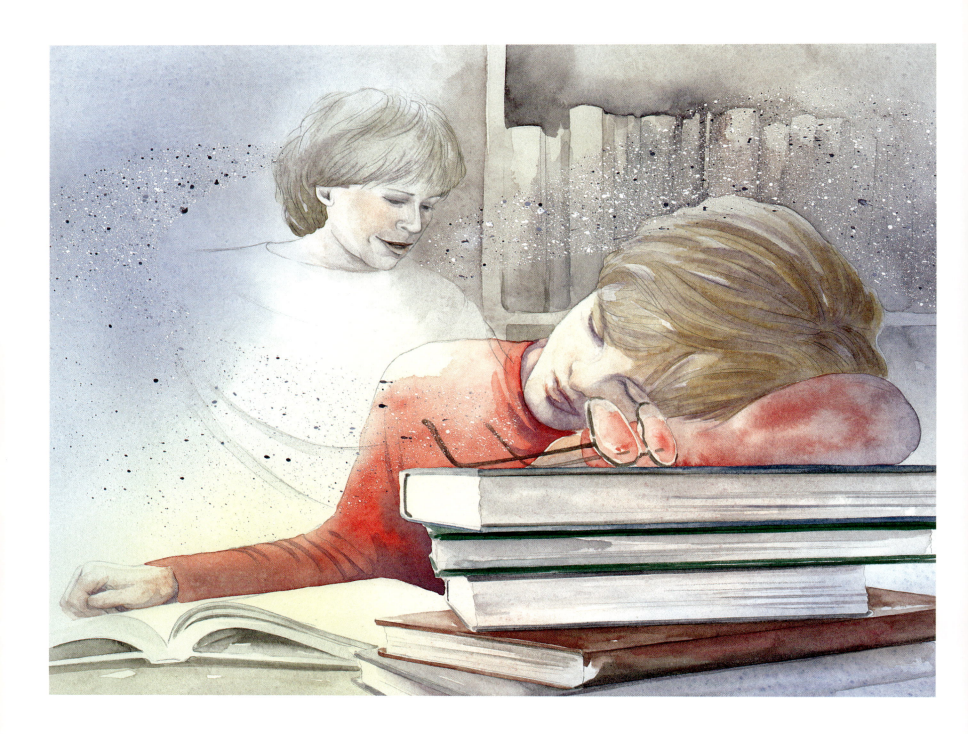

Sometimes she fell asleep at her books. When she did, she dreamed of Mommy's lullabies. Often she dreamed of Mommy whispering, "I believe in you, Katie Lynn!"

Now Katie works in the hospital where she was born. She helps heal the sickest, tiniest preemies. She loves being with the babies!

Sometimes she finds a baby who needs something special. When she does, she bundles him up, sits with him in the rocker, and strokes his face.

"Little baby, your name is Christopher. I believe in you, Christopher!" Then, in a soft, sweet voice, Katie Lynn sings a song her Mommy taught her when she was little:

Sleep, my child, and peace attend thee,
All through the night;
Guardian angels God will send thee,
All through the night;

Soft the drowsy hours are creeping,
Hill and vale in slumber steeping,
I my loving vigil keeping,
All through the night.

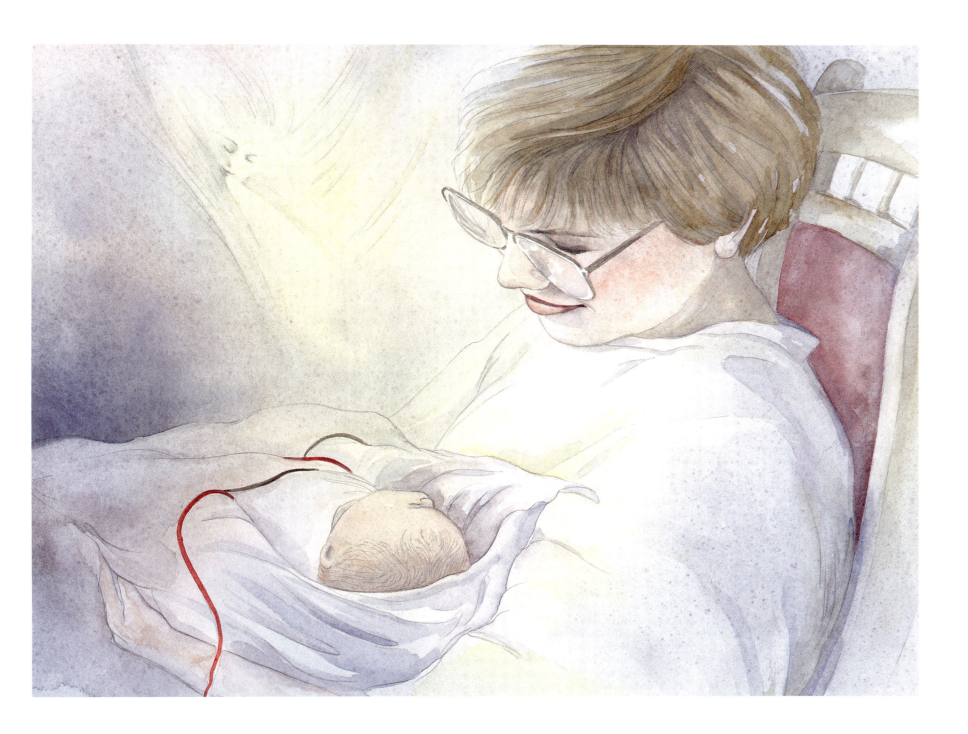

> *"Truly I tell you, just as you did it to one of the least of these who are members of my family, you did it to me."*

The great physician Lewis Thomas called medicine "the youngest science." The youngest branch of the youngest science *is neonatology:* the study of the disorders of the newborn.

Thirty years ago, a two and a half pound preemie had less than a fifty-fifty chance of survival. Medicine had neither the knowledge nor the tools to help. Now, most babies that size do wonderfully well.

They do well because of new insight and new technology. Researchers have provided ever improving solutions to the medical problems of prematurity, such as temperature control, breathing, feeding, and fighting infection. Still, these tremendous advances are only part of the story.

Years ago, parents were not allowed in newborn nurseries. Lights were bright and alarms loud. Babies were handled only when necessary. My mother and father did not get to hold or even touch my preemie sister Sara until the day she left the hospital—seven weeks after she was born.

There were good reasons for those rules. Touching the infants could agitate them. Parents might pass infection to their babies. Lights and alarms stayed on so that no problem would be missed. Doctors and nurses practiced the best medicine they knew.

The babies, however, taught a still more excellent way.

Little ones have more energy for growing when they are not stressed by alarms and bright lights. Sick infants get better faster when their loved ones visit. And Mommies and Daddies long to hold their babies.

Preemies should always be handled with great care. There are times when they must not be disturbed. But even the sickest, tiniest preemies soon need gentle snuggles and sweet caresses, just as they need food, and water, and the air that they breathe.

Nurses and doctors learned these lessons from thousands of real-life Katie Lynns. The old rules fell away. The nurseries were transformed. In neonatology, the "youngest science" is reconciled with an ancient truth: all God's children need love.

Many wonderful people–patients and parents, teachers and students, colleagues, friends, and family– helped make this book possible. Thank you all!

We are grateful for the generous cooperation of Meharry Medical College, Metropolitan Nashville General Hospital, Clarksville Memorial Hospital, and Vanderbilt University Medical Center.

Special thanks to our families for their encouragement, patience, and love.